Inflammatory Enemy: Living With Vasculitis

Mark Ingram

ISBN: 9798884960114

Preface

Don't call me a victim. I'm not a victim. A victim is someone who feels they are oppressed or suppressed; who feels they have been wronged, injured or falsely blamed. To identify as a victim you must feel anger, hurt or helplessness. I do not feel any of those emotions.

Sure, I've met people who made it their mission to cause me harm both physically and mentally, they've tried to damage my life by lying, spreading malicious rumours, and seeking to impede my progress through vindictiveness, but none of them have, nor shall they, ever succeed.

For as long as I have my wits and a pen in my hand I will never be a victim, and those that seek to make me one will themselves at some point suffer from all the injustices that they seek to rain down on my head.

Welcome. Firstly I'd like to express my gratitude to you for purchasing this collection of my poetry and prose, which documents my diagnosis and journey with a condition known as Vasculitis. The profits from the sale of this book will go to Vasculitis UK, an organisation dedicated to funding research and providing education and support to sufferers of Vasculitis.

Vasculitis is classified as a rare disease; there are 18 known types all with different symptoms and treatments. It's also incurable and if left untreated potentially life-threatening.

My particular type is called large cell vasculitis and affects the vessels surrounding my heart. My red cells eat away at the vessel walls causing inflammation of the cell walls, and if particles become detached it can cause clots to block off the blood supply to my heart and other vital organs. It's a genetic condition and though I was officially diagnosed in June 2023 it had been within me for the previous 62 years. I just didn't know about it.

Looking back I had been having flare ups for at least 20 years; debilitating fatigue, severe dizziness, pains in my head and armpits, and I had been off sick a couple of times for periods of up to 6 weeks. Although my GP practice had not diagnosed vasculitis they had suggested various conditions, including vertigo, viral infections, stress, and inner ear issues, but I had no specific diagnosis except that my blood tests were way out of the normal range. One GP did tell me that my immune system was compromised but didn't know why. They thought it was most probably as a result of a viral infection.

Friends, colleagues (I work in a hospital) and family were sympathetic and concerned, at least initially. After a while some of them were unkind to say the least, both to my face and behind my back. I was often in pain, extremely fatigued, and frightened because I didn't know what was wrong with me and the clinicians didn't seem to be any more informed than me.

I began to get stressed, anxious, and suffer with low moods and was prescribed antidepressants. This way of life continued for many years until I began to experience excruciating headaches, and in May 2023 my wife insisted that I sought a second opinion. Acting upon this suggestion I attended a new GP practice and saw another doctor. After taking a history of my symptoms he referred me immediately to Burton hospital.

Over the next few weeks I had a multitude of scans, blood tests, and a temporal artery biopsy before the Rheumatology consultant informed me that I had Large-cell Vasculitis. It's also referred to as Large-vessel Vasculitis (LVV). It's rare to have the condition in the area that I have it (my heart), and although my initial reaction was one of relief at having a definite diagnosis I was also concerned due to the area affected and the knowledge that without treatment my life expectancy was somewhat compromised. My symptoms of fatigue, headaches, pins and needles, severe pain in my armpits, loss of balance and feelings of nausea persisted which my consultant resolved through my medication.

I had to start using a walking stick to mobilise, and at times I was sleeping for very long periods of time. Gradually as my steroid therapy and other medication kicked in I began to feel more like a human being, and my daily life improved.

Throughout this period of time I kept writing, sometimes with anger, at other times with dark humour, and as I reflected I tried to express a sense of optimism. I performed my work at poetry evenings, and in partnership with my wife Carol arranged a fund raising evening in September 2023 which raised a significant amount for Vasculitis UK.

Amidst all this turmoil my wife Carol has been amazing and utterly selfless. She has been with me every step of what has been a very difficult and harrowing journey, and I will never be able to thank her enough for her love and unstinting support. My family and close friends have also been so supportive and loving. I am a very fortunate man indeed. Of course my GP practice, Queens Hospital in Burton, and the Rheumatology Team have all been supportive and utterly fantastic. Without them who knows where I would or wouldn't be?

This book contains a selection of poems that have that I wrote during the period from the onset of my vasculitis up until very recently. I hope you buy it (or have already bought), read it, and enjoy it. All the money raised will be donated to Vasculitis UK. I also hope to perform a selection of these poems as part of a poetronica duo called Apple Venus with my friend Russell Smith at fundraising events around the UK.

I appreciate you reading my intro and I hope you enjoy the rest of the book.

Peace and Love
Mark Ingram
March 2024.

This collection is dedicated to all Vasculitis sufferers wherever you are.
You are not alone

Mark
March
2024

Contents -

On The level
Neither up nor down
Extremis no likey
I would like to be level
Neither tyrant nor clown
Plateau unlikely
Not angel nor devil
It's a lifelong ambition
Being boring appeals
A face in the crowd desired
A break with tradition
Just to know how it feels
I'd like a complete rewire
So what does it take?
How to proceed?
Is there a simple solution?
Or I am cursed to remain?
Forever the same?
A one-man internal contusion.

Codeine Crash
To ache is human
To float divine
Awake but not woke
I'll put a spoke in your throat
Cry me a raincloud
Call me a psycho
I may be a cripple
But I've still got my mojo
More front than BoJo
Bigger arse than JLo
Who knows what I know
Not many El Loco
Temazepam come down
Amytryp to my loo
No need for a gee up
I'm coming for you
I'll CBD you later
Good night and God Bless
My life is enlightened
Yours is a mess.

I Know The Void
I live in extremis
I feel through other people's pain
I recoil from sunshine
I dance in the rain
I've only known suffering
I'm damaged by joy
I know the void

Plague is my dowry
Pestilence my gift
Criticism provides succour
Betrayal a lift
I walk over hot coals
A precocious humanoid
I know the void

Misery is welcomed
Disease an old friend
My hatred will haunt you
Right thru to the end
I'll laugh at your deathbed
I embrace schadenfreude
For I know the void.

Coma
It's warm here
No fear?
All is clear
In a coma

You can't hear me
But your voice is clear
I am aware
In a coma

Warm sleep
Cold existence
Reach out to me
In a coma

Contemplate tomorrow
There's joy
There is no sorrow
Peace is a coma.

Tension
Tension, such tension
Keep job?
Early pension?
Sickness!
Uncertainty!
What will change?
Is it cancer?
Is it real?
Am I a chancer?
What if inconclusive?
Then what?
A fraud-No
Its real, I feel it
I'm scared
Because I'm not frightened
Tension, and this is the tip
But what of, the tip of the iceberg
That sinks my Titanic?

Infected Song
You can't catch it
You've just got it
You can't cure it
You've just got it
They can miss it
It's undetected
It's not a virus
But I'm infected

Chorus: I'm infected x 4

You can't see it
But you feel it
There's no reason
You've just got it
It comes and goes
You can't be protected
It's in my genes
Yes, I'm infected

Chorus: I'm infected x 4

It never sleeps
When you got it
Dormant but still alive
When you got it
An ever present foe
To be respected
It's a ticking bomb
When you're infected.

Eaten From The Inside
Blood flows thick
Cells collide
Eaten from the inside
Immunity has no place to hide
Eaten from the inside
Cell walls corrode
Good cells die
Eaten from the inside
Temple throbs
Pain like fire
Eaten from the inside
Body won't move
Constantly tired
Eaten from the inside
Limbs don't function
Cos your brains hot wired
Eaten from the inside
Shooting pains
From side to side
Eaten from the inside
Scared to sleep
In case you die
Eaten from the inside.

Dissonance As Beauty
Grab dissonance by the horns
Shake it till you don't know you're born
Celebrate your uniqueness
Flaunt your utter freakiness
Push your individuality
Celebrate personality
Feel no shame
No ones to blame
What will be will be
You be you
I'll be me
What makes me feel
What makes me suffer
Will only serve to make me tougher
This disease that lives within me
Will soon become a friend and set me free.

Blessed

Go back, go back; return
To when you were born, unlearn
All the things that you see
Which stops you from being who you want to be . . .
You were innocent, you were pure
But now you're afraid and unsure
Take time to think and rearrange
It's always a good time to change
Night time terrors
Human errors
Words that wound
Looks that kill
Heart grows weary and
Feels the chill
Take time to think
Reflect and rest
It's then you realise
That you are blessed.

Never Too Late
Eat your teachers
Absorb their knowledge
Then spit out the bones
Take the digested knowledge
And use it
Don't lose it
Or their deaths will have been in vain

Drink the blood of the monarchy
The plasma will entitle you to a life of luxury
Reject the rest its acidity
Will blur your lucidity
And enhance your stupidity
To a quite an alarming level

Cannibalise the captains of industry
And watch as they gorge on each other's bloated carcasses
Celebrate as they realise they are infecting each other
With very bite
Corpulent cadavers, rictus grin
They died happy so it's a win-win situation

All life is made for consumption
It says so in Farmers Weekly
It must be true
It has to be true

Have no compunction
About human consumption
It's the logical conclusion
The only solution
To world-wide pollution

When the beasts of the field are no longer
Allowed to thrive and grow stronger
Its then that I know through all my pain
I'm just a cog in the cruel food chain.

Alive Again
Went to sleep sucking lemons
Woke up eating a peach
Everything that once seemed impossible
Now somehow seems within reach
The storm that had once gathered
Is now soft summer rain
I'm alive again

The frowns on the people's faces I've met
Are replaced by warm happy smiles
Life now feels so wonderful
It no longer seems like a trial
Positivity pours from my soul
Creativity swims through my brain
I'm alive again.

A Clear Out Is Required
Your heart is open
Your mind is closed
Failure to explore the truth
It's a one way road

Too many friends
Clogs up your loyalty glands
Pressure to please
Pressure to cede

Your eyes are open
But feelings are stunted
Trapped in a fools meditation
Your reactions are blunted

These friends
Check out their motives
Pressure to coalesce
More inevitably means less

Your diary is open, your options few
Too much confliction, you need a page a minute to view
Jettison the unwanted guests
Your house will be in order

Are you a friend in need?
Or are you a friend in greed?
Cut your losses, wield the axe
Trust your instincts, cover your tracks.

Cirrhosis Of The Heart
Don't know where the end is
Don't know where to start
I've a fractured sense of justice
And cirrhosis of the heart
Can't see straight for looking
My brain is blown apart
Morally I'm bankrupt.
I've cirrhosis of the heart
My nerves are beyond shattered
Blood pressures off the chart
A temper like a typhoon
And cirrhosis of the heart
Doctor says its terminal
I say he's a tart
I can live for years and years and years
With cirrhosis of the heart.

The Art Of Being
You can't be looking over your shoulder
Forever fearful of yesterday
Tomorrow's going to happen and that's a fact
Don't let preconceptions get in the way
Or judge yourself on mistakes you've made
Look forward and smile, and in a while
All those bad memories will fade
Once you accept that you are gonna die
No way out, no reason why
Then you can be more self-forgiving
And get on with the art of living.

Bald Tyre
Fractured?
Beyond help?
Past not present
Future blank
Bombs away
Crumbling but not antiseptic
Useless interred

Airborne pariah
Death in the skies
Save the excuses
Let the money talk
It speaks more truthfully
Of your actions
Than a thousand press conferences

You want it
You got it
But at what price?
The power behind the throne
Justified by history
While the future bleeds
Recurring oceans of blood

What chance of peace?
When tomorrow is held hostage
By the horrors of the unknown.

And It's A Wonderful Life
Looked around and counted my blessings
There were more than one or two
Happiness is never far
From a heart that loves it's true
Music regenerates a poisoned soul
Sunny side up; that's me
It's a wonderful life so live it to the full
Let music set you free.

That That Is Not
Your lifestyle is fauxganic
As buoyant as the Titanic
Behaviour cruel and manic
Designed to instil panic
Send the masses frantic
On both sides of the Atlantic
It's rape, but he calls it tantric
It's true, but perhaps pedantic
It's life but not as I know it
I'm strange but not afraid to show it
Not scared although I may blow it
Pass me the ball and I'll throw it
Terrified of your own reflection
Self-serving is your protection
I won't vote in your rigged election
I'm relieved by your smug rejection
Don't drown in your own sorrow
Don't steal my lines and don't borrow
I'll happily plough my own furrow
You stay today, I'm gone tomorrow.

Why?
It takes a lot
That's all I'll say
Trust has to cut both ways
Paranoid never no not me
You're out to get me, wait and just see
Best to quit whilst I'm still behind
Shattered dreams of a broken mind
Sick to the pit
Cut to the quick
It's all turned to shit
It's making me sick
No need to deceive
No use for pretence
It's best that you leave
There's no self defence
You took what you wanted
Then put out the fire
I stand here affronted
You stand there a liar.

Ears Don't Blink #2
Ears don't blink
They know the truth
A conduit to your brain
You can close your eyes
You can close your mind
But ears don't blink

Ears don't blink
So stop and think
Your words can wound and scar
Your mouth may forget
And your conscience may be blind
But ears don't blink

Ears don't blink
They're not a text
A Facebook meme or curse
When all else is gone
Words still remain
And ears don't blink.

Under Your Pillow
Tell me your secrets
Don't hide away
What's new to your heart
At the break of the day?
Is fear on the horizon?
Is your life filled with sorrow?
Leave it all behind under your pillow

Hell waits for no man
Heavens a chancer
The future's a mystery
And you don't have the answer
When there's no horizon
When happiness feels hollow
Look for a clue under your pillow

A turn of the card
There's a fortune to be made
The devil calls the tune
And deals the ace of spades
Too late to alter your fate
There will be no tomorrow
Hidden under your pillow.

Safe And Sound
Everybody needs a place
A place that's warm and safe
Away from daily rough and tough
All the pressure and mucky stuff
For some it's the family hearth
For others it's solitude
A bustling pub, a country walk
Meditation or a chance to talk
Wherever it is and in whatever form
I hope you all find it and feel safe and warm.

Bleed Through Dreams
Carnivore carrion
Carnival of corpses
Creation becomes catastrophe
Carnal crimes condemn me

Breath thru blood
Burnt and broken
Base and brittle
Behemoth beast

Abeyance through suffering
Angst for alternative
Alive to agony
Attraction by alchemy

Doom and despond
Dark and dismal
Dread to dream
Death by damage.

Carnival Of Leeches
Elected by trusting fools
Believe your own bullshit
Suck the truth out of diction
Pervert the law to fiction

Play to win at any cost
Serve yourselves till all is lost
Justice too far out of reach
In the carnival of leeches

King and country pledge
No depths that you won't dredge
The vulnerable left to die
Let the bodies pile high

Fatal flawed decision
And you're above suspicion
Let us live the crowd beseeches
Die fools die, intones the carnival of leeches

As you romance with your whore
Bodies pile up by the score
Another senseless bungle
Just send me to the jungle

No time to say goodbye
Families left to cry
We'll fight em on the beaches
Gloats the carnival of leeches

Locked down, locked up, locked out
There's a truth somewhere no doubt

But no justice for the masses
The fucked up working classes

As leeches leer and booze
The sick are left to lose
Our good health betrayed by rhetorical speeches
Left in the hands of the carnival of leeches.

Magma In My Veins
Feel the rush
Feel the fire
Head to toe
Brain hardwired
Heart beat quickens
Stomach sickens
Nerves twitch
Vision thickens
Balance thwarted
Speech aborted
Veins pulsing
Logic contorted
Blood rushing
Fear gushing
Sleep stifling
Pulse pushing
Heart blurring
Speech slurring
Walk wobbling
Stomach churning
Pain persisting
Is this existing?

Life's Simple Dilemmas
Open your mind and follow your dreams
All may not be as it seems
You think yourself in control
But in that twilight world of surrender
All that lies beneath the subconscious
Comes out to play

Is the past a place of memories sweet
Warm and comforting a safe retreat
Or does it force you to recall
The things you did and said
That can no longer be repressed
When Morpheus is at play

Are you hung up, repressed, depressed?
Or are you happy, optimistic and fully blessed?
Does fear consume your night-time?
Does ambition fuel your dreams?
Does lucidity bring you solace?
When everything is not as it seems?

Grey To Blue (For Carol)
Too many years of conflicting voices
Muddling my mind, restricting my choices
Opinions at work, in papers, on TV
Stifled my thinking, I was lost at sea
But all that changed when I met you
My life was transformed from grey to blue

Lived in a world of industrial smoke
My head and my heart were beginning to choke
Consuming a lifestyle that leads to distress
My body was broken, my mind in a mess.
But now my outlook has a healthier hue
My life is changing from grey into blue

Life's full of contrasts, a yin and a yang
My music is sweeter than the sad song I sang
The future looks clearer, the outlook is bright
I'm out of the darkness and into the light
And I owe the change all down to you
For bringing my world from grey into blue.

Hope In The Future
I can hear silence
I can feel peace
Love permeates my soul
Turn off tunes and feel the power of serenity
Forget the past
The future can wait
Live in the now
Be at peace
All souls are born equal
All babies are pure
Hate is an instrument
Used by the wicked
Dressed up in lies and deceit
Designed to create misery
Seek freedom and hatred will shrink
Show love and hatred will die
Utopia is within our grasp
Banish borders, inter uniforms
They are designed to make us feel fear, inferior
No human is on a higher plane than another
Renounce all that causes division
Turn your back on servility
Rise up with love
Rise up as one beautiful organism
Speak of peace and war will surely end.

Nice Try

It's not a competition
There's no selfless act of contrition
You only learn to be yourself
By embracing the act of living
There's a space for commas and question marks
But the full stop finally comes around
When you accept that you can't change what has gone before
With both feet on the ground
You can live your own life story
But it takes courage to write it down
Too many hire a ghost writer
Who comes in from out of town
Interviews are permitted by sycophants and fools
In an attempt to paint a picture of innocence and cool
But I won't write a story, a fable, or a parody
I'll tell it like it is and I'll state it proudly.

21st Century Schism
What was that you said?
What was that you tried to say?
A noise, an empty void
Intent but with no purpose
Sentences with form
But no meaning
Promises made to be broken
Words said but unspoken
A cliche ridden catastrophe
The tracks of your tears
Trace the path of your fears
Rain until the clouds are empty
Cry until your eyes go blind
No sun will curse your withered bones
No pillow for your head to rest upon
Just stones, cold thrown stones
Is this the world we created?
The harlequin once sang
No, it's the world we decimated
As the bells of Sodom rang.

Manifesto #3
Wakey Wakey!
Rise and shine
C'mon in, the water's fine
Be productive
Don't waste time
Use it wisely
Don't use mine.
Lick the bowl
Taste the air
Eat your fill, but just your share
Think of others
Not just yourself
Do not covet personal wealth
Use words sparingly
Weigh up their worth
Criticise warily
Words do and sometimes hurt
Mean what you say
Then deliver
Don't sell your sibling down the river
Never sleep when your enemies are awake
Make vigilance a habit
There's too much at stake
Treat animals as equals
Not as slaves or as food
Disregarding nature
Will do you no good
Make humility a virtue
Plan where you're going
Embrace and accept your mistakes
It helps your progress, it keeps growing
Love with your whole heart
Hold nothing back

Don't stretch yourself taut
Give yourself slack
Be as kind to yourself s you are to
Neighbours and relations under attack
Don't be pious
Or quick to judge
Don't be too frivolous
Don't be a drudge
Here ends my manifesto
A prayer if you like
And last but not least
Check the brakes on yer bike!

Not Dead Yet
I'm broken, but not busted
I'm ring worn, but not rusted
I'm hurting, but still hoping
I'm weary, but still coping
I've cried, but I'm still laughing
Not working, but still grafting
I know hate, but I still love
And when it comes to push and shove
I'm still worthy of your money if you fancy a bet
I may be down, but I ain't dead yet.

Acknowledgements
Thank you to Langton Medical Centre, Queens Hospital
Burton, Dr Das and the Rheumatology Team, Gurvinder Singh,
Jane, Pat and Cliff at Unison, Richard – physio, Michala Dytor,
Delves Baptist Church, Ian and Jill Giles, Russell Smith, Bob
and Dylan for cuddles and fuss, my dad, my sister Sara, my
bro-in-law Andrew for love and support, my three fantastic
kids Jack, Niamh and Holly (and Rhian and Mitch) for always
just being there and loving me no matter what, to Meek for
editing and contributing to this book, and finally, to my
beautiful wife Carol without whom I would have cracked up.
Your never ending love is the greatest gift I have ever had.

Mark
xxx

Mark Ingram

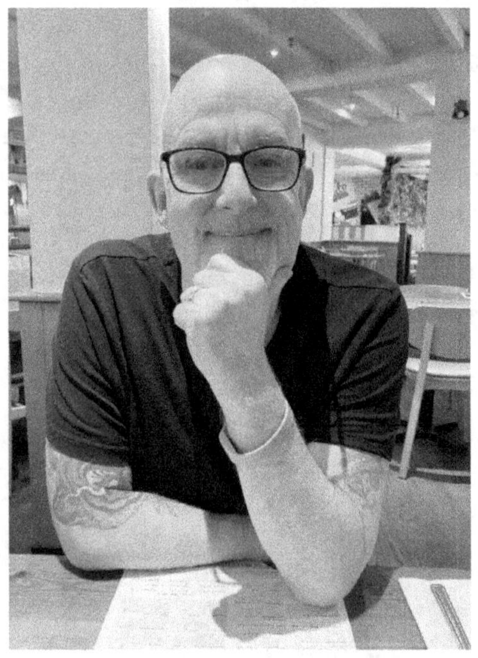

Mark Ingram is 63 years old, lives in Lichfield with his wife Carol and their two cats Bob and Dylan. He has large cell Vasculitis!
Mark writes prose and poetry and performs in an electronica duo called Apple Venus with Russell Smith.

Publisher

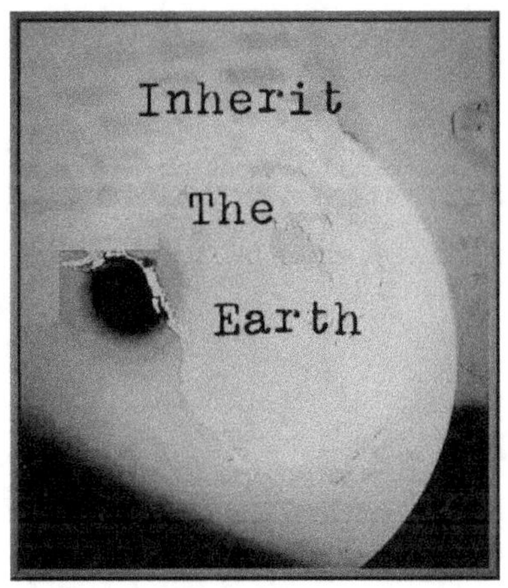

inherit_theearth@btbtinternet.com

Notes